The Survivor in Me:
8 Steps to Healing

Lisa A. McDonald, M.Ed.

Scripture references noted "ESV" are taken from the Holy Bible: English Standard Version. Copyright © 2001, Wheaton: Good News Publishers. Used by permission. All rights reserved.

Scripture references noted "KJV" are taken from the Holy Bible, King James Version. Public Domain.

Cover designer: Veronica J. Bernal
Logo: Design by Lik
Photographer: JCP Photography
Publishing consultant: Obieray Rogers (www.rubiopublishing.com)
Writing coach: Cynthia DeVese

ISBN 978-0-578-60716-0

To contact the author, please visit www.lisaamcdonald.com

This book is dedicated to my role models and heroes from day one—DeWitt Sr. and Ella P. McDonald. I love you both!

ACKNOWLEDGMENTS

Thank you, Lord, for this amazing opportunity to share my story with the world! I'm grateful for the support of and encouragement from those who gave me their time, energy, and assistance for the two years I pondered writing this book.

I thank God for my supportive husband, Omar C. McDonald Sr., as it couldn't have been easy listening to my story repeatedly, and then continually reading my rough drafts. To my three sons, Quincee, Omar Jr., and Christopher—thank you for allowing me to work even though it meant taking time away from you to meditate and write.

A sincere thanks to my parents and siblings for being so supportive and encouraging. I appreciate them standing in the gap for me when I was too weak to do it for myself.

I am so grateful that my sister, Cynthia, took me under her wing as an author and assisted and encouraged me every step of the way.

A special thanks to my surrogate daughter, Maurissa, for always being there when I needed her the most, without hesitation.

Thanks to Christine Lynch, my therapist, and Roxanne Shante (Lolita Shante' Gooden), my friend, for your willingness to read my manuscript and for writing such encouraging words.

I appreciate my friend, Dr. Chanda Elam, writing the Foreword and endorsing the book.

FOREWORD

The Survivor in Me: 8 Steps to Healing is the personal story of Lisa McDonald, who overcame life-threatening health challenges while raising a newborn baby and starting a new life on her own.

This book serves as a guide for women who have faced obstacles in their lives and overcome them, one day at a time. Lisa shares with the reader the feelings and emotions of a young mother newly diagnosed with breast cancer, while coping with a failing marriage. Her faith, courage, and strength—displayed throughout the book—can help any woman who has just been informed of a life-changing situation and who needs encouragement to keep fighting. While Lisa did not know what the outcome of being diagnosed with cancer would be, she knew that she had to continue to fight for herself and her son. In many circumstances, women have to be the parent, the protector, the family support, and the breadwinner—all rolled up into one. The question to ask yourself is: what happens when you're challenged to your breaking point and have to rely on family and friends to make it over the hurdle? This book gives you an opportunity to understand Lisa's deepest thoughts and the hardships she endured in a way that's never been portrayed before.

As a child of a woman who lost her battle with breast cancer, this book has helped me through my healing process. I was able to understand the journey from a survivor's point of view: the fear, the recovery, the remission, and the need for continual support of family and friends. All too often in the black community there is a silence (almost shame) about dealing with pain, illness, or death; which then leaves the next generation to start the process all over. Lisa McDonald gives a blow-by-blow account of the process of diagnosis, surgery, recovery (short term), and continual monitoring of a woman who survived and beat cancer.

Chanda Elam, Ph.D.
President, Elam Consulting Services

Contents

INTRODUCTION

I grew up in a small city in Ohio along Lake Erie called Sandusky, in a middle-class family headed by my parents, Dewitt and Ella. I was the youngest of 5 siblings: Sharon, Loretta, Dewitt Jr., and Cynthia. Our parents were hard workers and excellent Christian role models, who stressed the importance of attending college and making something of ourselves.

I was an above-average student, who traveled from seventh through twelfth grades with the same 20 students. We were the gifted and talented class. I was popular in school, and sports helped me interact with the rest of the student body.

As the youngest sibling, I was the last to leave my parents' home for college. I attended Bowling Green State

University's (BGSU) main campus in Ohio, the same school my siblings attended. My major was Biology/Pre-med. After I graduated with my bachelor's degree, my plan of attending medical school was short-lived; so, I began taking classes to obtain my teaching certificate. Because I wanted to work with children, I became a science teacher and taught for five years. During that period, I completed my master's degree in Educational Leadership, Administration, and Supervision.

Like most people, I've had my fair share of ups and downs, drama and trauma, highs and lows. And, like most people who are survivors, I tapped into the inner strength that wasn't evident until needed. When I look back on my life, God has always been there for my family and me. I've been in challenging situations since I was a child, and God has never failed to see me through.

I've often thought of what it means to be a survivor. According to dictionary.com, a survivor is a person who survives, especially a person remaining alive after an event in which others have died; the remainder of a group of people or things; and a person who copes well with difficulties in their life.

As I pondered the subject of survival deeper, I realized that I would need a certain mindset, skills, and attributes to overcome whatever I faced. I focused on eight attributes that helped me cope, heal, and move forward throughout each situation I encountered. The following steps are what helped me:

1. *A Positive Attitude*—I had to focus on the good and not the bad. I had to get a grip, pick up the pieces, and move forward in a positive manner.

2. *Mental Toughness*—Once broken, I had to utilize specific tools to survive and live a better life. For me, this meant prayer. However, it also meant seeking help from my personal spiritual source (mine was and still is God), a licensed therapist, and a life coach.

3. *Motivation*—I had to push myself from within, accepting unconditional love from family and friends. It also meant being willing to give back to others.

4. *Work Ethic*—I had to keep a strong work ethic and do my best until the job was done.

5. *Adaptability*—I developed flexibility to rapidly changing events. I realized it's okay to change your routine to maintain survival.

6. *Determination*—I embraced a strong sense of purpose. I never gave up even when the outcome seemed negative.

7. *Perseverance*—I maintained persistence in difficult situations. I never lost the will to fight.

8.   *Resilience*—I adapted the ability to recover from difficult situations gracefully.

While experiencing the life-changing events described in this book, I applied the above attributes. I managed to come out of potentially harmful situations with positive results and an uplifted mindset that changed my life for the better. *The Survivor in Me: 8 Steps to Healing* may help you do the same.

− 1 −

FACING THE UNKNOWN

My first husband proposed on the morning of Memorial Day, May 26, 1997. We had lived together from December 1994 to February 1997. I moved into my own place in February because we weren't getting along and we argued almost daily. I felt our relationship was not moving forward, so I broke up with him and moved into one of my parents' homes to have a fresh start. The time apart gave us a chance to see if we wanted to be together. By April, he was practically living with me. My parents—Rev. Ella and DeWitt McDonald, Sr.—are Christians who don't believe in "shacking up" before marriage. My mother regularly spoke to us about getting married, if we wanted to be together.

We were engaged for 3 months when he started to complain about feeling sick at work. I told him that he was probably dehydrated and needed to drink more water. This went on for 2 weeks, and I suggested that he go to the doctor. Around the same time, I noticed that I had missed my period; because my cycles were irregular, I wasn't alarmed. I had begun taking classes to get my master's degree from BGSU and was teaching science at my high school alma mater. The stress of it all could have caused my irregular cycle. A week later, I went to the doctor and discovered I was pregnant. I didn't say anything at first because I was in shock. I called my fiancé at work and told him the news. He was so excited, and I was silent. He asked what was wrong, and I told him that I didn't know if we were ready to have a baby. I also thought what my parents would say about us having a baby out of wedlock. Then I thought, well, we're grown, employed, and engaged. None of that mattered now; we needed to prepare for the baby's arrival.

We bought a new home in November 1997 and welcomed our new baby, Quincee, in 1998. We were happy and kept our original wedding date of August 8, 1998. Our wedding day was beautiful and included all of our family and friends. We honeymooned in Cozumel, Mexico, and the Grand Cayman Islands. When we returned, things were going well. A month later, I received news that would have a dramatic impact on our lives.

My mother-in-law called and said that my husband's grandmother, who raised him and his sister, had been shot in broad daylight while sitting in her chair watching television. She said that some people were outside of their apartment complex shooting; it appeared to be a stray bullet and, more than likely, gang related. I felt like I stopped breathing for a second because I knew this news would devastate my husband. I couldn't tell him while he was working, so I called and told him we needed to talk. I asked him to come straight home after work.

When he got home, he sat in the family room and waited for me. I decided to tell him straight out because there wasn't going to be an easier way. He sensed that something wasn't right, so I told him what happened. He said, "huh," fell to the ground, and immediately started to cry. I tried to console him, but nothing was helping. I knew that to him he had lost his mother, the one who raised him. We waited for a couple of hours before he called his sister and then his mother. We traveled to East Chicago, IN, where he was from and where his grandmother's funeral was held. This event changed our lives forever. He wasn't the same person and started to seem distant toward everyone.

When we returned home, his sister called and spoke to him about their mother. She had nowhere to stay, so we moved his mother into our home. She would keep our baby while we both worked, but because she was depressed, I'd take him to daycare some days. It worked out for a short time. In October 1998, my husband began staying out later and drinking more. I encouraged him to get help, but he didn't feel like anything was wrong. One night he stayed out past 2:00 a.m., and I went looking for him. When I found him, he had a female in the car and was dropping her off. This was the beginning of the end of our relationship.

We didn't talk for 2 weeks. I couldn't get over the incident and told him that we needed to go to counseling. He kept saying that he didn't want anyone in his business. I struggled to stay in the marriage because I could no longer trust him. I had a feeling that he had more infidelities. Of course, he denied everything, but my woman's intuition kicked in. I would hear about him in the streets and decided to give him an ultimatum: Either we were going to find new jobs, relocate, and start fresh, or we were going to get divorced.

The remainder of 1998 and 1999 was a challenging time for us being a young married couple with a baby. I continued pursuing my master's degree, taking care of our baby, and working fulltime. This was an extremely stressful time for me, but I didn't realize how much until Quincee and I got into a terrible car accident in the spring of 1999, coming from BGSU's main campus. I either fell asleep at the wheel or blacked out from exhaustion or stress. I lost control of the car, crossed into the opposite lane, and hit a utility pole. The whole front of the car was pushed up to my lap. This could have broken both of my legs. When I awoke, all I could think about was if my baby was okay. By the grace of God, I was able to get out of the car, go around to the back door on the passenger side, and get my baby out of his car seat.

As I held Quincee tight, I heard people talking to me, but I couldn't understand what they were saying. The voice that I did understand was my dad's. My father was traveling from the same direction coming from a small town named Fremont where he owned property. He came back to the scene after passing us and called in the accident, not realizing it was us!

The next time I woke up was in the hospital. I had fractured ribs and other scrapes and bruises, but nothing life-threatening. My baby didn't have a scratch on him! When my parents came to the hospital, Dad said the car was totaled and the way the car was crushed, no one would believe that anyone survived. God was watching over us and didn't allow any hurt, harm, or danger to silence us. He had a divine plan for my life! My husband wanted me to delay my master's degree to relieve some of the stress. I mentioned this to my mother, and she said, "If you know like I know, you better not!" Those few words meant a lot. I understood that I needed to persevere through that dark time to see the light at the end. On August 7, 1999, I graduated from **BGSU** with a master's degree in educational leadership and supervision.

In 2000, my husband took a new job with Ford that was 40 minutes from where we lived, but 15 minutes outside of Cleveland. I told him that I would look for a new teaching or administration position and began applying in the summer of 2000. I interviewed and was offered an assistant principal position with the then Cleveland Public Schools in January 2001.

We agreed to start looking for a house closer to the Cleveland area. We never moved; so, in November 2001, I decided to pack Quincee's and my things and move into an apartment outside of Cleveland and down the street from the school where I worked. My husband wasn't happy about my decision and filed for a divorce. I was okay with the filing because our marriage had been over for months. When I received the paperwork, I got an attorney. A few days after I signed the papers, my husband called and said that he didn't want a divorce but had filed because he wanted us to move back to the marital home. I told him I wasn't moving back, and that I wanted to move forward with the divorce. He was reticent, as if he didn't expect my reaction.

* * *

WHILE WAITING FOR the divorce to become final, I met someone special and began a new relationship.

On April 11, 2002, my partner noticed a lump in my breast. More curious than frightened, I examined myself and discovered not one but three lumps! I wasn't sure I wanted to know what they were, but my partner encouraged me to have them checked as soon as possible. The next day, I called my gynecologist for an appointment and was brought in for an emergency appointment the same day.

Many thoughts were going through my mind; it was hard to stay positive. When the nurse called my name, I felt like I was going to pass out. When the doctor entered the room, he immediately started asking questions about my health and my family's health history (this is important to remember). The doctor gave me a breast exam, felt the lumps, and told me that he was sending me to the hospital where I would get a mammogram and needle biopsy of the areas. At this point, I didn't know what was going on and decided to trust that the doctor would take care of everything.

I didn't call anyone to be with me at the hospital, so I drove there in a daze. A nurse was waiting for me upon arrival and took me to the preparation area. I had the mammogram and returned to the room to wait. The doctor came in and did the needle biopsy, which consisted of him taking a sample of cells or fluid from the lumps inside my breast to determine the status. There was a little discomfort with this procedure.

I was nervous when the doctor and the nurse left the room with the samples; they returned, saying that I would need to have an ultrasound. The doctor couldn't see much on the mammogram because the areas appeared to be too dense. Again, not fully understanding what was going on, I continued to let them proceed with the ultrasound.

After the ultrasound, I was told to get dressed and wait for the results. I waited for over an hour, growing more anxious and nervous with each passing moment. When called, I walked toward the doctor's office with my life flashing before my eyes. I sat down, expecting to hear the words, "No cancer." I held my breath when the doctor came in, releasing it only when he said that everything came back okay, and I didn't have cancer!

I was happy to hear this news. I left the doctor's office, praising God for His blessings! I immediately called my mother and told her about the lumps, the testing, and the results. She praised God with me and asked when I would have the lumps removed. I grew quiet and admitted that I hadn't thought about having it done. My mother was insistent that I have the lumps removed and not leave them in my body. I agreed and told her I'd have the procedure.

— 2 —
ROUND ONE:
THE REMOVAL

My soon-to-be-ex-husband was continually calling and wearing me down about giving our marriage another chance. He wanted us to move back to our home in Sandusky. I finally agreed to move back in June 2002 after school was out.

Being away gave me time to heal the hurt I felt in our relationship, but it also made me feel distant from him. He had been patient with me. After being back home for over a month, I still couldn't be intimate with him. That's when I knew for sure our marriage was over. We spoke about how we felt about each other. I knew it was difficult for him to hear that I loved him but that I was no longer *in* love with him.

I had been looking to build a house 25 miles outside of Cleveland in Streetsboro. My college roommate, her husband, and their children had built a house there, and I liked the area. I also knew that they'd be a great support for Quincee and me. After finalizing plans and making an initial down payment, the contractors broke ground in late July 2002. My final walk-through and closing were scheduled for November 2002.

* * *

I RELUCTANTLY SCHEDULED surgery for November 11, 2002. When I arrived at the outpatient surgery center in Sandusky, I had a positive attitude. I was encouraged by my previous diagnosis that I was fine and that this was a simple surgery to remove the lumps. The surgeon who was to perform the procedure was the father of one of my high school classmates. He and I talked before the surgery, and I felt relaxed and less stressed.

Because the lumpectomy was outpatient and I wasn't in much pain, I was able to drive to Cleveland for work the next morning. Determination fueled me to move forward and stay positive because I had to close and move into a new home to begin a life without my ex-husband.

My realtor called the day after the procedure to tell me the closing would be on November 29, 2002, as scheduled.

I was so happy, feeling like I could conquer the world, and nothing could upset me at this point. I remember feeling tired with some pain, but I still maintained a positive outlook knowing that I'd be getting off work soon. After picking my son up from preschool, I could go home, relax, and take some pain medication. Little did I know the next phone call that I received would change my life.

Since I traveled to and from work every day for 75 minutes each way, I listened to gospel or smooth R&B music. This was a way to calm and relax my mind from everything that I dealt with during the day as a vice-principal at a middle school in inner-city Cleveland. On my ride home, I received a call from the surgeon. He asked me if I could talk and if I were in a safe place. I told him yes, although I kept driving. He then said that the pathology of the mass removed the day before was malignant—cancerous! My whole body became tense. I heard the doctor say that he had already spoken to doctors at the Cleveland Clinic and arranged for me to meet them. He said that my initial surgery to remove the areas around my nipple and areola where the lumps were found was scheduled for Wednesday, December 4, 2002.

I was stunned into silence. The doctor asked if I had questions; I uttered "no" very softly as tears ran down my face and neck. Everything he said afterward was a blur. My 31 years flashed before me. I cried like a baby all the way home and spoke to God as I'd never done in my life! I asked the Lord to heal me and give me understanding. I asked God to let me live long enough to see 4-year-old Quincee grow up. All I could think about was my son and how I didn't want to leave him until he was fully prepared to take care of himself. I promised God that I'd never take people or things for granted again! My last statement to God was that I would never ask, "why me?" again, because why not me?

God spoke to my spirit and assured me He had a purpose for me, although I wouldn't understand it now. I was halfway home and couldn't cry anymore. It was as if God Himself had wiped my tears away! I felt a presence come over me that I'd never felt before, a feeling of being held, protected, and strengthened at the same time. A level of peace entered my mind that I couldn't understand, especially considering the new prognosis my doctor gave me. When I arrived in Sandusky, I was able to pick up my baby from preschool, go to the grocery store, and go home to prepare dinner.

I called my parents and shared the news with them. My mother immediately started to pray for God to heal me. She told me not to worry because God had the last word. As my mother prayed, I could hear my father on the other phone affirming the prayer and praying to God on my behalf. I told them that I'd cried all the way home, spoke to God, and that I was okay.

I asked my parents not to share the news with my sisters because I wanted them to hear it from me, so they'd know I was okay. This was a test of me being able to stay positive, upbeat, and strong while having to tell the family that I was in the biggest fight of my life. We were on a conference call when I shared my diagnosis with my sisters. Indeed, God doesn't put more on us than we can bear. While each sister reacted in her own way, I reassured them that I was going to be okay.

My mother informed my brother in prison about my situation, and I was able to speak to him a few days later. He was concerned but positive that everything would be all right.

I chose not to share with a lot of people what was going on, so I only told close family and friends. I also shared the news with my boss. I didn't want anyone feeling sorry for me or continually asking me about my situation. I didn't want people treating me like I was contagious. I had many mixed feelings and emotions, and all I could do was pray. I knew I needed to stay positive and continue my routine as much as possible before and after surgery. I continued to work until the day before surgery. I've always had a great work ethic, but this was different. I *needed* to continue working and staying busy so that I wouldn't fall into depression.

I had a lot of packing to do and only a week to prepare for the move from Sandusky into our new home in Streetsboro before surgery. I was able to gather a few friends who helped me pack and move in a week. I closed on my home on November 29, moved in on November 30, and was at the hospital for surgery on December 4! I had so much support from my family and friends, and I thank God for them all.

− 3 −

MENTAL TOUGHNESS

I never thought about my mental health being in jeopardy throughout dealing with the cancer diagnosis. When I went to my appointments at the Cleveland Clinic, I was offered counseling services but never accepted them. I had and still have a strong faith in the power of prayer, so I knew that was what I needed the most to keep me mentally strong. However, there were days I felt broken, sad, and lonely, like no one would understand how I felt because they hadn't dealt with the same issues. I was blessed to have praying parents who instilled in their children that God had to be the head of our lives, and that prayer would help us through anything and everything!

My parents came to stay with Quincee and me the day before surgery. My mother cooked some of my favorite foods. She prepared fried chicken and collard greens because I had to stop eating at a specific time, and she wanted me to eat a good meal. I had to be at the hospital by 6:00 a.m., but I couldn't sleep all night. I laid in bed, trying to keep my mind from thinking negative thoughts and praying that surgery would go well. We were up by 4:00 a.m., and left my house by 5:00 a.m., because it would take at least 30 minutes to get to the hospital.

When I arrived, I was taken to registration and then for pre-surgery prep. The entire time I prayed that everything would be okay, and that God would work through the doctors, nurses, and support staff who would be in surgery with me. After prep, I was taken to a room where I was able to see my parents, my baby, and my significant other before surgery. My mother prayed, and I knew God was there with me because I felt a peace and calmness come over me.

When I was wheeled into the operating room, the breast surgeon, plastic surgeon, 2 anesthesiologists, 3 residents, and 5 nurses were waiting for me. Each introduced themselves and stated the job they'd perform during surgery. I thought to myself, God, you know how to show up. You sent a lot of people to make sure the operation would go well. After the lead surgeon explained what was going to happen during surgery, one of the anesthesiologists put a mask over my face, and I was out like a light.

After 8 hours in surgery and 2 hours in recovery, I was taken to my room where my parents, baby, significant other, siblings, and close friends were waiting. The lead surgeon, a resident, and a nurse came by and shared the best news I could have received; they were able to remove all of the cancer! I was weak and in a lot of pain, but I was happy to hear that fantastic news. I cried tears of joy and kept saying, "Thank You, Jesus!" I stayed in the hospital for 3 days of observation and was released on December 7 to return home.

God indeed places people in our lives for different reasons and seasons. When I came home and found that the new and old furniture had arrived and been put together, I knew my partner had made it happen. He was incredibly supportive throughout this time in my life. I am forever grateful and appreciative for all that he did to make my move and recovery successful and smooth.

— 4 —

MOTIVATION

Recovery went well at home, but I was bored. Winter break for students was December 23, 2002 through January 3, 2003. I was motivated to continue recovering so that I would be able to return to work after the break. I missed engaging with the students and staff.

When I returned to work on January 6, everyone was happy to see me, and I was glad to see them. Being around people with positive energy helped me to fight through the pain I was feeling. It was also great to be working again so that I wasn't sitting around, always thinking about my situation. I slipped back into my routine of going to work, picking up Quincee, cooking dinner, and preparing for the next day.

I was scheduled to begin chemotherapy in February 2003. I didn't know the dynamics of taking chemo, but I knew it would lessen the chances of my cancer returning. I was motivated to get through this life-changing moment, so I began to read and research on my own. My oncologist told me that I'd have 4 rounds of chemotherapy. I wanted to continue working, so I opted to go on Friday so that I'd have the weekend to recover before returning to work on Monday. My chemo was scheduled for every 2 weeks on a Friday. My parents came to my house the night before and took me to my appointments. They stayed in the room while I was taking the chemo. Again, counseling was offered, but I declined because I had great support.

When I arrived at the Cleveland Clinic for my initial chemo treatment, I met with the oncologist. He explained that I would receive the chemo drugs intravenously and that it would kill any remaining undetected cancer cells and keep new cells from forming. He also shared how I would feel and the side effects. In my mind, I thought that I wouldn't be able to eat at all and that I'd lose too much weight. He told me that I would feel okay but that I wouldn't be able to eat solid food that first day after the treatment because it would cause me to vomit. He also told me that since the drugs were red, there was a strong chance that I wouldn't want to drink anything red, my taste buds would change, I wouldn't want to eat right after the treatment, and I would possibly feel nauseous.

The oncologist further disclosed that after my second round of chemo, I'd start to lose my hair, have a weird, chalky taste in my mouth, my fingernails and toenails would become discolored, and I'd be weak and tired. I asked for clarification about my hair, and he explained that I'd lose the hair on my head and all body hair, which included my eyebrows. I listened while he continued to talk and felt overwhelmed by the information. I had to be hooked up to a machine and receive the chemo for 3 hours without a break. He had the nurse take my vitals and give me what looked like an IV. She hooked the drugs onto the IV, asked was I comfortable, and told me that the drugs would feel cold going through my veins at first.

As I laid on the hospital recliner bed, I kept reminding myself to stay positive because this wouldn't last forever. I was praying, my parents were praying, and they kept me motivated by being there and supporting me. After my treatment, I felt a little tired but not sick to my stomach. The nurse offered me graham crackers, and they tasted delicious. I drank some water, my vitals were retaken, and I was released to go home. When I got there, I went straight to bed. My mother made chicken noodle soup from scratch for me to drink the broth since I couldn't have solid food.

When Quincee arrived home from daycare, we were happy to see each other. He got in the bed with me and cuddled. As I held him, I knew that God was watching over us. Knowing that I had to live for my son motivated me to follow the doctor's instructions and eat better so that I could return to work to support my baby and myself financially.

— 5 —

WORK ETHIC

I returned to work after receiving my first round of chemo, and I felt good. I thank God I was able to continue my work responsibilities without limitations. The 2 weeks between each chemo treatment did me a world of good, even though I knew what was in store after my second round.

The same procedures were followed to administer my chemo, but something was different the next day. When I started combing my hair, some of it came out on the comb. Because God had already let me know that everything was going to be all right, I understood that this was part of the process to heal.

I've always had long hair down my back, so I called my sisters. I told them that I wanted them to come to my home the following weekend to cut my hair. I wanted them to be a part of that moment and to know that I was genuinely okay with losing my hair. I also wanted to cut my hair on my terms and not let it fall out in patches.

My sisters came the following weekend and took turns cutting my hair. It was an emotional time for all of us. It couldn't have been easy knowing their baby sister was fighting for her life. As they tried to hold back their tears, I remained strong and reassured them that I was feeling fine, and I was going to be okay.

I had bought a few wigs earlier, so I tried each one on, and they decided which looked best on me. I returned to work for the first time wearing a wig. The color and style were close to my hair, so it didn't attract too much attention. I didn't know anything about wearing a wig, but I discovered quickly how hot and itchy it was for me. I found that I needed a human hair wig and not a synthetic one. That day on the way home from work, I stopped at the wig store to purchase a human hair wig.

I was excited to finish chemotherapy in late March 2003. As usual, my mother made chicken noodle soup. I thank God because I didn't experience any vomiting after each round of chemo. Since it was my last day of chemo, I wanted to eat the noodles and chicken and not just the broth. I ate too much soup that evening and paid for it overnight! I was vomiting all night and had horrible stomach pain. As I gripped the base of the toilet with my hands, I prayed and asked God to once again see me through this and promised I wouldn't detour from the doctor's orders again.

My oncologist gave me a final check-up and the best news ever: There was no cancer in my body, and the chemo hadn't done any damage. He told me that I'd be seeing the radiation oncologist because I would start my rounds of radiation in 3 weeks.

–6–

ADAPTABILITY

I knew my lifestyle had to change. I was going to have to eat healthier and exercise to get stronger and feel better. My mental health was getting better—my divorce was final in early April 2003—and I was about to start 6 weeks of radiation for 30 minutes every day, except for Saturday and Sunday. I researched radiation and the side effects, but nothing could have prepared me for the reality.

I met with the radiation oncologist in mid-April 2003. He told me I'd experience some fatigue and some skin irritation or itching. I'd be able to work but needed to schedule treatment for the end of the day, if possible. The students were dismissed at 2:30 p.m. each day, and I had to pick my son up by 6:30 p.m., so I scheduled treatment for 3:30 p.m.

I had a great support system of friends. Lori and Joelle lived in the same new housing community. We had met during our freshman year at BGSU. Lori and I were roommates, and Joelle was always with us. I met Michelle while I was an assistant principal at Nathan Hale Middle School in Cleveland. I met my daughter-like student, Maurissa, when she was a 12-year-old attending Whitney Young Middle School, my first assistant principal job. Each of these women was instrumental in helping me to adapt by assisting with Quincee and doing everything to make my life easier. The transition from chemo to radiation was uneventful because my stress level was low due to the support.

I started radiation on a Monday in April 2003. I had to remove my shirt and bra only. The oncologist explained that the radiation would be targeted to kill cancer cells in my right breast, which meant that the side effects from the radiation would affect my skin on, underneath, and around my right breast. I was instructed to lie still for 30 minutes because the radiation needed to hit the targeted treatment area to be effective. During my first treatment, I didn't feel anything. I laid on that hard table and prayed to God to see me through the next 6 weeks. After my initial treatment, I felt fine, put on my clothes, and drove 40 minutes home to get my son. I was so thankful to God that I didn't feel tired.

The first couple of weeks were similar; by the third week, I began to get tired and sore around my breast. My right breast was burned and raw on top and underneath. As the weeks went by, my skin began to darken. There were days the pain was unbearable, but I fought through and kept going to work and to my daily treatments. I had to adjust my sleeping position from my stomach to alleviate the pain from my right breast. By the last treatment, I was so sore and in pain that all I wanted to do was take some over-the-counter medication and go to bed, but I had to keep moving.

After 6 weeks of treatments, I saw the radiation oncologist the following week. He stated that he didn't see any cancer from my scans. He reiterated what I needed to do to ease my pain and heal in hopes that my skin would lighten and become as healthy as possible. One of the things that I used was ice in a plastic bag covered with a towel. This, along with Tylenol®, did wonders and helped me to sleep through the night. I wanted to celebrate the end of radiation treatments, but I was in too much pain. I had to pull it together because my journey was far from over.

Two weeks after radiation, I met with my oncologist, and he introduced me to a pill—Tamoxifen®—that he was confident would keep cancer from returning. He told me it wasn't a 100% guarantee, but it had done wonders for patients who had taken it under his care previously. The doctor told me that the side effects were that I wouldn't be able to have any more children because I would experience menopause very early. I'd also have night sweats, headaches, fatigue, mild insomnia, depression, hair thinning, and mood swings, which all sounded worse than chemo and radiation! Once again, I had to rely on my faith and know that God was working through the doctor to get me well. The last thing the doctor said while writing the prescription was that I had to take the pill every day for 5 years. I went to the pharmacy, got the prescription filled, and headed home. I began taking the medicine the following morning.

It didn't take long before I started experiencing many of the side effects discussed earlier. The most memorable were the night sweats. I'd wake up most nights drenched in sweat as if I had run in a marathon! I'd get up, change my bed, and attempt to go back to sleep, which didn't happen often. I figured this was my time to talk to God and let Him know that I wasn't questioning Him but only wanted a sign that I was going to be all right.

I was still dating my significant other, and he encouraged me to stop wearing the wig. He told me almost daily how beautiful I was without it. I stopped wearing the wig in late 2003. My hair was like a newborn baby's—really fine and short. I went to the barber and had him line me up. I felt so free without the wig, and I loved rocking the short style.

In August 2005, I began a new job with the Streetsboro City Schools, only 5 minutes from our home and across the street from Quincee's school. I needed this break from driving into Cleveland every day and the stress of being in an urban school. That's not to say the new school didn't have any stressful issues, but they were different and manageable. The latest move gave me time to look into opening a small business that I could do from my home, so I took a tax preparation course in September 2005. My decision to accept the new position and open my tax business were some of the smartest decisions I made while taking the Tamoxifen®.

I continued to get better and returned to the Cleveland Metropolitan Schools to work in 2006 as a principal. I met a lot of people who I took on as tax clients at that time and managed to become close friends with Chanda and Resa. I worked at the high school level from 2006 until 2010. My last dose of Tamoxifen® was in May 2008. The entire time I took the drug, I didn't experience being sick one day. I didn't miss a beat. Now was the time for my body to recover fully.

My last assignment was a PreK-8 school on the West side of Cleveland. I stayed there from 2010 until 2013, when the unexpected happened.

–7–

ANOTHER CHANCE AT LOVE

In June 2011, I was invited to attend a friend's daughter's high school graduation party in upstate New York. One of my best friends, Tammy, drove with me and our other best friend, Shana, met us there. I've known both young ladies since we were kids, and we've managed to keep our close relationship throughout the years.

The party turned out to be a lovely event, but we had to get some sleep before returning to OH the next day, a Sunday. The following morning, some of the ladies were discussing shopping in the city because it would be a new experience. Tammy and I were preparing to leave when we were asked to stay. It didn't take much convincing for us to take a road trip to New York City (NYC) to shop.

About 8 of us piled into 2 vehicles and headed out. We had a 3.5-hour trip, and we hadn't confirmed hotel rooms for the night. We ended up stopping at a gas station/restaurant area for a restroom and food break after a couple of hours.

As we were leaving the restaurant, a man spoke to me saying that I was gorgeous and had nice feet. I thanked him and kept walking until he asked me to slow down. He asked for my name and where I was from, and I asked him the same. When he told me that his name was Omar and he was from NY but lived in NJ, I knew we'd never connect. He said that he could tell I was in a hurry but asked for my number. I told him I didn't give my number out. Instead, I asked for his, thinking we'd never speak again. Omar gave me his number and told me that he got off work the next day at noon and looked forward to talking to me. I smiled, got in the truck with my friends, and left. We reached NJ and stayed in a horrible hotel 20 minutes outside of NYC. It was a long night, but we got up early, ate breakfast, and went into the city.

Most of the group had heard about the Macy's store on 34th Street but we didn't know how to get there. There was so much traffic with people driving recklessly and horns blowing loudly until reaching Macy's almost became an afterthought and not a reality. We were lost, and someone suggested that we call the guy I met the day before for directions. I thought this was a bad idea because I didn't want him thinking that I wanted to talk to him. I finally accepted my friends' urgings and called Omar. He asked where we were and then gave great directions that led us straight to Macy's door. Omar and I continued to talk while we were all walking from the parking garage and into the store. When we got inside, I thanked him and told him that I'd call him later. The store was huge! We had fun shopping, and everyone was grateful that Omar helped us.

From that day on, Omar and I talked almost daily. He seemed friendly and was easy to get to know. He loved to talk but had limited time because he was working a lot of hours, but he often called during his breaks. Our conversations flowed, and he always asked about me, my son, and our well-being.

In August 2011, Omar asked if he could fly me to NY to visit him. I agreed, and he bought a ticket for me for Labor Day weekend. Our visit was wonderful; neither of us wanted the weekend to end. When I thought about what had occurred, I couldn't believe I had flown to another state to visit a man whom I'd only seen once before that weekend.

Omar and I continued to talk frequently, and he made plans to visit me in October 2011. We had fun during his visit, but he had to go home for work. Omar called me on his way back to NJ and said that he'd found the ideal halfway meeting place for us: Penn State University. For the next 6 months, we took turns traveling to see each other. When we couldn't go the entire way, we met at the halfway point in PA.

In February 2012, Omar brought Omar Jr., to OH to meet me. He and my son got along fine. After a few more occasions of all of us spending time together, Omar asked if Quincee and I would move to NJ with him and Omar Jr., with the understanding that we'd get married in 2013. We had fallen in love and knew that we wanted to spend the rest of our lives together, but I struggled with leaving my job, family, and independence. After many discussions and prayer, I decided to take a chance to see if this would work. I spoke to Quincee, who was okay with the decision.

Omar and I agreed that we'd move in the summer after school was out. I told him that I'd look for a job in NJ. If I couldn't find one by the time school started, I'd return to my school, work during the week, and fly back to NJ on the weekends. This meant that I needed to decide where Quincee was going to school for his freshman year. Being an educator, I knew the importance of making sure he was stable for his high school years. He'd need the best education possible without the interruption of transferring to a different school.

Omar and two of his younger brothers, Michael and Lance, came to move us on June 28, 2012. This was my first big move out of OH. I was apprehensive, but I also felt I was making the right decision for us. My friends Resa and Maurissa helped us move, although it was Resa's birthday. We loaded everything into a U-haul and 3 cars.

I had acquired a certificate of eligibility from the state to become an administrator in the NJ school system. By August 2012, I hadn't signed a contract of employment and returned to my job in Cleveland. Omar asked if Quincee could go to school in NJ so that I wouldn't be stressed with the transition. I agreed and flew back and forth every weekend, coming home on Friday and leaving early Monday morning. This continued until I got a job with the Newark Public Schools in 2013.

On Friday, May 17, 2013, I flew back to NJ on an early flight. As usual, Omar picked me up from the Newark airport, and we went to dinner at one of my favorite restaurants in Queens, NY, called Dallas BBQ. After dinner, we went to the Brooklyn Bridge Park in Brooklyn, a beautiful park that we had visited many times. It was my pre-birthday, and I hadn't seen my boo all week so, of course, I was looking cute, wearing very high heels. We walked around the park, and I told Omar that I needed to sit down but I wouldn't tell him my feet were killing me! He agreed but wanted to walk to another area of the park, although it was getting late.

When we arrived at the other area, we sat on the bench and gazed at the stars while I took my shoes off. Omar began telling me how much he loved me and didn't want to live without me. He told me I'd made him and his son's lives better. Then, he got on one knee. I asked what he was doing and urged him to get off the dirty ground. He pulled out some roses and a beautiful blue box and asked if I'd marry him. He opened the box, and all I could see was lots of sparkle on a gorgeous ring. I started crying because the proposal was unexpected. Omar impatiently asked, "Well?" and I said, "Yes!" I gave him the biggest hug and kiss ever! I was the happiest woman in the world! He said, "Happy birthday, Princess," and when I looked at my watch, it was 12:15 a.m., on May 18, my birthday. Omar had timed everything perfectly.

We were married at a courthouse in a small rural town in NY. Our families were happy for us, but my mother thought that we should get married in a spiritual setting surrounded by close family and friends. We renewed our vows during a beautiful ceremony in OH.

In mid-October 2013, I noticed I hadn't had my menstrual cycle and told Omar. I felt okay, although I should've had my cycle 2 weeks prior. We bought a home pregnancy test, the kind with 2 tests inside, and immediately took the first test. It took a while before it turned, but it read positive! I told Omar it had to be wrong because I couldn't have any more children because of the Tamoxifen®, so we took the other test. It turned positive quicker than the first one! I told Omar I was going to make an appointment with a gynecologist, and he jokingly said, "You're pregnant. There's no need to go to the doctor." I refused to believe this, so I went to see the doctor.

I was confident the doctor would confirm that I wasn't pregnant. So, while they took blood and ran tests, I knew the results were going to be negative. The doctor came in with a look of happiness on his face. I said, "I *knew* I wasn't pregnant," and he said, "No, ma'am, you are *definitely* pregnant!" I sat in disbelief and insisted on a second opinion. The doctor assured me that the blood test was one of the most effective available.

I left the office with mixed emotions. I was scared because I didn't know what the future would hold. I was happy because God had shown me at that moment that He can exceed any expectations that I could have for getting pregnant. And, then, the devil raised his ugly head. "Girl, you know you're too old to be having a baby. You're 42. Who's going to take care of it?"

I called Omar. He was excited about the news but could tell by the sound of my voice that something was wrong. He told me not to worry; that everything would be okay, and this would be our miracle baby. We bought a beautiful home in PA in May 2014 to accommodate our growing family. We moved in early June to prepare for our new arrival. I had an uneventful pregnancy and delivered a handsome boy, Christopher Quincee.

– 8 –

THE UNEXPECTED

In August 2014, I was asked to become the principal of the Barringer High School S.T.E.A.M. (Science, Technology, Engineering, Arts, and Math) Academy in Newark, NJ, because the principal of one year had been fired. I was honored to be asked, but I was on maternity leave until November 2014 and wasn't looking to become the principal of another school. I wanted to start a life-coach and consulting business and quit working in the public schools altogether. However, the opportunity was presented, and after talking with Omar and meeting with the superintendent, I accepted the position.

My first day on the job was August 25, 2014. I reported to the district office and was informed that I was no longer going to Barringer but to Weequahic High School. The school was scheduled to close, but the community fought and won to keep it opened. I was confused but reported as instructed. Upon arrival, I was disturbed to see a huge fence in front of the building, causing the school to resemble a prison. An immediate goal was to remove the fence before the students and staff arrived in early September.

Another priority was to bring some people to this school that I had built good working relationships with at the previous school. I was only able to hire 3 people because the other positions were already filled since schools were scheduled to open in 8 days. I prayed for God to give me the strength to prepare for a smooth opening because there were many obstacles in the way.

The first year was very challenging. The school had been scheduled to close, and the previous principal was on medical leave. Staff jobs were in jeopardy because the district wanted to close this school for low performance and enrollment. There was poor communication between the assistant superintendent and the vice-principals, and the students were feeling uneasy because they didn't know who to trust because of the high staff turnover. I spent the first year working on listening, learning, repairing, rebuilding, and restoring.

Our second year was a continuation of the first, but the light was beginning to shine. It was evident that the culture and climate of the school and the attitudes of the students, staff, and parents were becoming more positive. Trust was coming back. Our attendance and performance test scores improved, and our graduation rate increased by over 5% within 2 years.

In the third year, we continued to gain momentum. We increased our attendance and performance test scores even more, and our graduation rate by another 2%. In 3 years, our graduation rate went from 66% to over 73%. We were proud of our accomplishments. Also, in the third year, our boys' basketball team made it to the state finals, and our football team was the NJ state champions. Many positive things were occurring, and we were moving upward.

Toward the middle of the school year, I began hearing rumors of being replaced by a male principal. The rumors continued throughout the rest of the school year. On graduation day in June 2017, the board chairperson told some staff members they'd have a new male principal the following school year. When they immediately shared this information with me, I was shocked! I couldn't believe this underhanded behavior was going on behind my back. The rumors were beginning to take a toll on me. I spoke to my boss the next day. He advised me to ignore the board because they were new and immature. He also stated that no one could fire me except him or the superintendent. I tried to hold on to what he said, even when the rumors persisted throughout the summer.

When I returned to work in early August 2017, I thought that everything was okay. I hadn't heard anything from my boss except to report to scheduled professional development, and the dates principals were to attend. My boss and I discussed bringing new programming to the school during one of the meetings because he thought my school would do an outstanding job.

In September 2017, students and staff came back to school, and we were looking forward to a productive school year. The rumors started to surface again, and I shared this with my boss. He told me to focus on the academics and to filter out the noise. I took his advice.

We had a great school opening; I was glad to see my students and staff in good health. Things were looking up for us. I was contacted by the Mayor's Office and told about an event they wanted to hold at our school involving some high-profile political people and former NBA player Shaquille O'Neal. The program was an opportunity for students to hear Shaq speak about the importance of staying in school regardless of obstacles. The event occurred in late September. At this event, a high-ranking school official told some of my teachers that they were going to have a new male principal by the following Monday. Of course, it got back to me. I reassured them that it couldn't be true because my boss hadn't spoken to me; plus, it was already the middle of the week. The following Monday came, and I was still the principal.

On Friday, October 6, 2017, my boss sent me a text asking if I'd read my email, which I hadn't. When I finally read my email, it said that I needed to report to a meeting with him and the human resources person to discuss my future with the Newark Public Schools. Soon after, I received a phone call from a union representative, who was also a principal. She asked if I knew what was going on. I told her I didn't. She didn't either and asked me to meet her 30 minutes before the meeting. We didn't know the nature of the meeting, so we entered blindly.

My boss began by saying that my school hadn't increased in performance for the past 3 years. He and I knew this wasn't true since it was in black and white on the New Jersey Department of Education's website. As he continued talking, instead of getting upset, I felt a calmness come over me as if Jesus was saying, "Peace! Be still. I've got you." I sat back in my seat and stared into space, knowing that all this was stemming from what I was told back in December 2016 about being replaced by a male.

When asked if I had any questions, I declined but offered a few comments. I told my boss that he could have moved me or terminated me back in June 2017 when I mentioned the rumors and what had occurred. I also let those in attendance know that I was aware they had already hired my replacement and knew who he was. They both looked shocked. My representative asked if I was ready to leave; I was but needed to get my things. I returned to the building after school was out to get my belongings.

Everything seemed off about this termination—how it happened and my union not knowing anything about it. I felt helpless and broken, but I knew that I had no choice but to fight.

$-9-$

DETERMINATION AND
PERSEVERANCE

I met with the union after discovering they knew nothing about my termination. We decided to file a complaint because I should have had tenure. Also, I hired a personal attorney to file a wrongful termination and gender discrimination complaint. We filed both complaints in late December 2017.

During this time, I applied for jobs frequently, but nothing was happening. I became frustrated, depressed, isolated, and couldn't sleep. I didn't want to go anywhere or do anything most days, so I stayed in bed while the baby was in daycare. I began to feel ashamed and embarrassed as if

I'd done something wrong. I prayed to God for help so that I wouldn't lose my mind. I needed to talk to someone and reached out to a licensed therapist. The stigma of disclosing that I was dealing with issues that were affecting my mental health didn't matter to me anymore. It was important for me to seek help and work to get mentally healthy for myself and my family.

Since I hadn't found employment during December, I decided to take a portion of my retirement money and start a luxury gifting business named Luxe and Love. A former colleague who also worked for the Newark Public Schools gave me the idea. We traveled to China in January 2018 and met with 5 of the manufacturers who were assisting us. I also started IMPAC Coaching and Consulting Group. I figured if I was going to invest in anything or anyone, it would be myself.

Meanwhile, both cases were moving forward. The Equal Employment Opportunity Commission (EEOC) began their investigation to see if my complaint had any merit for wrongful termination and gender discrimination. In August 2018, after investigating for 8 months, the EEOC found in my favor. Because the district didn't enter conciliation with EEOC and my attorneys, we received a right to sue letter that allowed us to file a formal lawsuit against the district as of December 2018.

Unfortunately, the tenure case wasn't decided in my favor because I only met 2 of the 3 needed criteria. I had my standard principal's license and more than 4 years with the district under my NJ license; however, I never received an evaluation from my boss. Because of that lapse, I didn't achieve tenure. (Obviously, something is wrong when a decision is handed down based on things that were out of my control.) My union representative and I were upset and wanted to appeal the decision. The attorney for the union felt that since the Commissioner upheld the decision, it was unlikely that it would be overturned.

That decision was a low point for me; but knowing the power of prayer and with the help of my therapist, I was able to rise above it emotionally. With everything in me, I had to fight once again as if my life depended on it. I was unwilling to give in to the fear of being ostracized or being isolated to conform due to lies and injustices.

– 10 –
ROUND TWO:
ROUTINE CHECKUP

The beginning of 2018 was the perfect time for me to invest in my future, especially since my career was ripped away from me overnight without warning. The trip to China to meet with manufacturers who helped in some of the designs for Luxe and Love Co.'s luxury gifting items was inspiring. I learned a lot about sourcing, retail, and the various grades of products. It was the opportunity of a lifetime to travel overseas and indulge in a different culture.

We did our first pop-up shop on March 25, 2018, at a salon in Orange, NJ. It was a success and we made $2,500.

This was confirmation that we were selling the right products. I worked hard to acquire everything needed to open a kiosk at a mall in Paramus, NJ, on April 16, 2018. The sales started off slowly the first day, but the second day and thereafter, the sales were good. I had 3 employees, and within the first month, I hired 2 more. Business was good for the first 3 months, and we were making a weekly average of $5,000. The initial thought was to do the kiosk as a pop-up shop for 3 months before moving to another location to do the same. I was working at the kiosk up to 6 days a week. On top of this, I was keeping up with inventory, ordering, scheduling employees, and taking care of all other business entities.

Needless to say, I was stressed out and knew that I needed a short vacation. In the middle of July, my husband and I left for Puerto Plata in the Dominica Republic to rest and relax. We spent the week basking in the sun, enjoying a couples' massage, eating amazing food, and rekindling our relationship. Even though I promised my husband that I wouldn't work, I found myself texting and emailing the employees to find out what was going on and the total of our daily sales. We didn't want the week to end, but we had to return home to our children and work.

When I returned to work, it appeared that everything was running smoothly until I started looking more closely at the business account. I discovered that the total monies that were supposed to be deposited each day wasn't correct. I called our eCommerce provider and found that we had been receiving chargebacks on the account that I had to pay back.

I was concerned and began my own investigation. It seemed that every time one specific employee worked, there were multiple individual purchases of over $200. The chargebacks were most of the purchases under this employee. The handwriting was on the wall, but I didn't want to believe that my top employee was running a scam on the business.

In early August, I called a meeting with all the employees and shared some of my findings. I had them sign an agreement that they would follow proper procedures and use the chip for each credit and debit card. If the card was swiped and the owner claimed they never made the purchase, an automatic credit was given to the customer by their bank. Employees were responsible to pay for the cashbacks if they used the swipe instead of the chip. This was a nightmare.

As I uncovered more information, I knew I had to involve the police. In September 2018, I filed a formal police report and within 24 hours a detective got in touch with me. He told me that they would pull video footage for the specific days and times in question, so I would have to supply that information.

A few days later, the detective contacted me. He emailed me photos that he retrieved from the security video. There were multiple pictures showing my employee sitting with 2 males while she was supposed to be working. Some of the pictures showed the men with business logo bags filled with merchandise. The detective thought it would help if I spoke to the employee. I attempted to get her to tell me what was going on, but she denied everything. I knew that I had to fire her.

The detective and I spoke again, and he decided to pick her up from the kiosk and take her to the station for questioning. She was video recorded and continued to lie about not knowing the men in all the pictures. She claimed they were returning customers. Something told me to check her Instagram account. I found that she was friends with one of the men, so I forwarded the information to the detective. As the detective dug deeper, he uncovered that it was a credit card scam that was being run in many stores throughout the mall. By this time, my business losses with merchandise and money totaled over $20,000! I fired her.

The detective explained that he wanted to get enough information on the men to arrest them. I questioned him about arresting my employee, but he didn't feel he had solid information that would stick. I felt hopeless. I couldn't believe that someone could steal from me, not have to pay the money back, and not get charged and arrested for engaging in criminal acts. The situation continued to go unresolved.

My spirit was broken, and I couldn't seem to recover from the loss quickly enough. I fired the other 2 employees and decided to run the kiosk myself. Of course, this pace wasn't sustainable for me because in November and December the mall was scheduled to be open 14 to 16 hours each day. I hired one of the employees back to help throughout the holidays, but we were overwhelmed. I made the decision to close the kiosk in December 2018. I was stressed out. I started getting bad headaches and feeling sick. It was time for me to take care of my health.

* * *

ON JANUARY 1, 2019, I resolved to take better care of myself. So, the next day, I scheduled and kept appointments with a new gynecologist and a new oncologist where I lived in Easton, PA.

My gynecological results came back normal. I had skipped a year without getting an annual exam, so I was thankful to God for the news. The oncologist scheduled a full screening of tests from head to toe at the Easton Hospital. I was back and forth for 3 days, getting an MRI, pelvic ultrasound, and a CT scan, to name a few. It was overwhelming, but I endured every test so that I could have peace of mind about my overall health.

My oncologist contacted me to come to his office the day after the last set of tests. He told me that I needed to get a biopsy because of 2 areas found on my left breast. The procedure required an operating room, so he had his scheduler make an appointment with the surgeon for the next day. I didn't know what to think or how to feel but knew that I'd been here before.

During my consultation with the surgeon, we discussed my previous battle with breast cancer in my right breast so that he could gain some insight. He explained that he was scheduling me for a stereotactic breast biopsy to look at 2 different areas in my left breast. Both areas were deep inside my breast, but one was thicker than the other. He added that both areas could be benign and that more than likely there was lots of scar tissue from my past reconstructive surgeries.

The following week, I had the first biopsy on my left breast. The procedure was different from the biopsies I had 17 years ago. I had to lay on a hard, cold table on my stomach with one breast extended through an opening in the table. The surgeon, radiologist, and nurse were present. The procedure was like a mammogram in that the nurse moved my breast into different positions and took pictures. I was awake the entire time as the surgeon talked me through what he was doing.

After the procedure, I went home and relaxed with pain medication. I was relieved that it was over, but then I began to stress about what the results could indicate. I knew that it would take a few days to receive the results. The not knowing was torture.

I called the surgeon's office after the third day because I hadn't received a phone call. The doctor was out, but the nurse told me that everything looked fine according to his notes and that I had an appointment scheduled for the following week. I was happy and relieved. I immediately called my husband and parents, and I texted my siblings and close friends that the areas were benign.

When I went to the appointment, the surgeon told me about the biopsied areas, showed me the X-rays of both areas, and confirmed they were benign. The dense area did show something, but the surgeon said I didn't have to be concerned because it wasn't cancer. He told me that he would see me in August for a checkup and to keep an eye on the dense area. He sounded very confident that I was going to be okay.

I left the office thinking I don't have cancer, which was great, but what was going on with this dense area? Then I remembered the doctor said he would check me again in August; prayerfully, that would be great news. The euphoria was momentary because when I returned home, I received a call from my oncologist saying that he wanted to see me the following day.

When I got to his office, I'd already decided to have a positive attitude because all he was going to do was reiterate the surgeon's information. The oncologist arrived, pulled his chair close to me, and said, "We need to talk about your results." He confirmed that the one area was benign, but the denser area was high-risk and required immediate removal. If I didn't get it removed quickly, it would turn into cancer and be more aggressive than my first battle, requiring at least 9 months of chemotherapy! I was stunned into silence. My doctor informed me that because he researches breast cancer, especially in younger patients, he knew what to look for when reviewing X-rays and other tests. The look on his face was a sense of urgency that I'd never seen from any doctor. He explained that he didn't want to scare me, but he had to let me know this was extremely serious.

I pulled myself together enough to ask why the surgeon said I was okay and would check me in August. My oncologist explained that the surgeon was using older methods of diagnosis. The surgeon didn't have pertinent knowledge about breast cancer in patients who had their first diagnosis and treatments before the age of 40. My oncologist is a researcher and had conferred with other research oncologists who confirmed his findings and beliefs. I couldn't stop thanking him for not sitting on information that could have potentially been detrimental to me. He asked if I wanted to move forward with surgery at Easton Hospital; I told him that I would return to the Cleveland Clinic.

I left the doctor's office in disbelief. I tried to get myself together, but I started crying and couldn't stop. I felt my whole world crumbling. The only thing I knew to do was start praying to God to see me through this situation like He did the first time. I called my mom when I got into my car. I told her what the oncologist said, and she immediately reminded me that God had me, and I was going to be all right. She was confident that God had seen me through my first cancer battle, and He'd see me through this, too. I left a message for my husband at work; he called me back within minutes. He was my rock and told me not to worry and that we would do whatever was necessary. He let me know that he would be there every step of the way.

I contacted the Cleveland Clinic the next day; my appointment was scheduled for the following week. The nurse requested that I bring all records, scans, and reports to the appointment. My husband, Christopher, and I packed our things and headed to OH. Quincee wasn't with us because he was in college and working. My stepson, Omar Jr., was finishing his senior year in high school, so he remained at home.

−11−

FEAR IS NOT YOUR FRIEND

On the morning of February 28, 2019, my husband and I traveled 6 hours to the Cleveland Clinic for my first appointment at the Taussig Cancer Center; my mother and my sister, Loretta, met us there. When I arrived, I gave the records, scans, and X-rays to a nurse via the receptionist. I completed some paperwork and waited to be called in to see the doctor. As I waited, feeling and looking fine with no pain in my body, I observed many people who appeared to be very ill. I began to call on the name of Jesus because I knew that whatever was going on inside my body, He would take care of it.

The longer I waited, the more nervous I became, and fear raised its head. I didn't know what to expect. We waited for more than 2 hours before I was called back. My mother went with me. The nurse gave me a robe and told me that the surgeon wanted to take new mammogram pictures. The procedure was slightly discomforting.

As the mammographer and nurse looked at the images, I could hear them conversing about the dense area in my left breast. I was told to return to the waiting area and that the radiologist would view the mammogram pictures. I was more nervous than before, and my mind immediately went to worst-case scenarios. My mother attempted to distract me by talking, but it didn't work.

The nurse came to get me and said that the radiologist was ready to speak to me about the results. The radiologist put the X-rays on the lighting machine so I could view them with her. She pointed out the area that was benign and then the dense area, which resembled thick tissue. She told me that she had spoken to the breast surgeon, and they agreed that another stereotactic biopsy of my left breast was needed to be sure of the area and to mark it in preparation for surgery. They wanted to do the procedure that day, and I agreed.

I had a 3-hour wait before the procedure, so we grabbed something to eat. My nerves were on edge, but I tried to act as normal as possible. I was happy that my family was with me.

We returned to the Taussig Cancer Center, and I was immediately taken for the biopsy. It was the same painful and uncomfortable procedure as before. As the doctor talked me through it, I asked the Lord for relief. It seemed like forever, but the procedure took about 40 minutes. I knew the pain was necessary to get an accurate diagnosis. The doctor was able to get 3 samples of tissue to send to pathology for review. The radiologist told me that I did a good job. The nurse cleaned me up, and I got dressed and headed to my next appointment with the breast surgeon. The surgeon's nurse took my vitals and asked about my family's history of cancer. This information was necessary for my records. The breast surgeon came in, greeted us, and reviewed my chart. He seemed positive and started by saying that the biopsied areas didn't look cancerous, but the tissue was being sent to the pathologist for a final review. I wanted my mind to be relieved, but it wasn't.

He asked if I had been given the BRCA genetic test. I said no. He explained that I needed to have the testing done to determine my susceptibility to other forms of cancer. If the test returned positive, then my children, siblings, and their children would need to be tested to see if they could be carriers. The doctor wanted me to get tested the same day after I left his office and arranged for me to have my blood work done.

Before I left the surgeon's office, he asked the nurse to locate the genetics counselor for a consult. The counselor explained that my blood would be used to run various tests on my chromosomes to determine whether I was positive or negative for the BRCA gene. It would take 10 to 12 days to get the results. After receiving the results, the breast surgeon and the plastic surgeon would know best how to proceed. I would be scheduled to come back to the clinic to receive my results and possibly be prepped for pre-surgery.

I remembered hearing that the actress Angelina Jolie had taken the BRCA genetic test, and she was positive. She chose to have a double mastectomy to lower her chances of having breast cancer. I now had to consider what to do if I were positive for the BRCA gene. Without hesitation, I'd have a double mastectomy to lower my chances of getting breast cancer again.

I left the doctor's office and went across the hall to have my blood drawn for the genetic test. It was a simple procedure, like having regular blood work done. I thought about what was about to take place, and instead of being fearful of the unknown, I was optimistic. At least I'd know what I was up against and how my future would look regarding breast cancer recurrence.

Two weeks after my genetics test, the counselor contacted me with the results. I was positive for CHEK2. My heart was beating so fast, it felt like it was going to come out of my chest! The counselor said that being positive for the CHEK2 gene mutation meant that I had a higher rate of recurrence for breast cancer, and an increased chance of getting other cancers like colorectal cancer. Upon hearing this news, I instantly knew that I wanted to get a double mastectomy. I didn't want to keep going through the not knowing when it would occur again.

The counselor asked about my siblings and said that it would be good for them to come to my next appointment to discuss the need for them to be tested. The information I received was overwhelming, but I knew that I didn't have time to waste. When I got off the phone with the genetics counselor, I immediately called my mother and texted my siblings. Even with this diagnosis, everyone was upbeat and encouraged me to stay positive and know that God was working things out.

The following week, my mother, my mother-in-law, and my sisters traveled to the clinic for my appointments. Since I had relayed to the genetics counselor that I wanted to get a double mastectomy, my appointments were scheduled with the breast surgeon, genetics counselor, and the plastic surgeon.

The first appointment was with the breast surgeon. My entire family was invited to come into the observation room with me. The doctor was pleasant, as usual. He reviewed my chart and started talking about the positive CHEK2 gene mutation. He said there wasn't a lot of information about this specific genetic mutation. What he did know was that it made my chances of getting breast cancer again higher, but not high enough to get a mastectomy. He stated that because the high-risk area was detected before turning into cancer, he would remove the high-risk tissue and the tissue around it. The doctor seemed confident that this procedure would have a good outcome, and my breast cancer recurrence would be lowered.

The doctor canceled my appointment with the plastic surgeon and said we'd revisit the mastectomy option later, if needed. I was glad to hear this information but eager to know when my surgery would be scheduled. While the doctor was talking, the genetics counselor came into the room. The doctor introduced him, asked if we had any questions for him, and then left the room. The genetics counselor went over the results from my genetics testing and explained to my mother and sisters that because I have the CHEK2 gene, it was a possibility that they could also be carriers. He gave them all the information they needed to share with their healthcare providers for genetic testing. The nurse came to escort everyone to the waiting area and took me to get pre-registered for outpatient surgery, scheduled for April 29, 2019.

When Omar and I returned home, I realized that Christopher's kindergarten registration day had passed. I contacted the school secretary, and she rescheduled me for the following morning.

−12−

RESILIENCE

While waiting for the surgery, I continued working my online retail business. I also received a consulting contract to do business with a school district in NJ beginning April 2, 2019. I stayed positive and started the work, knowing that there was a chance that I wouldn't be able to finish by the deadline of June 9. I was determined to be strong and push through. The school would be on spring break during my surgery, so I kept the faith that I'd be able to return soon after to complete the work.

I got up at 3 o'clock in the morning on April 27 to pray for safe travel and success for my surgery. I specifically prayed that no cancer would be found. I also wanted to make sure that I had everything needed for the trip to Cleveland. I knew that my husband was tired of making the 6-hour drive, but he never complained. Omar picked up his mother and aunt the night before so that they could travel with us. This would be a great support for me, but also for my husband and our son, Christopher.

Since the clinic was close to downtown Cleveland, my oldest sister reserved rooms at a nice hotel where we stayed until the morning of the surgery. My in-laws had never been to Cleveland, so they got a chance to enjoy good food, shop, sightsee, and go to the casino located on the lower level of the hotel. Participating in these activities with my family helped relax my mind and kept me from thinking so much about my upcoming surgery.

Monday, April 29, came quickly. I had to be at the Cleveland Clinic by 6:45 a.m. Instead of reporting to the surgical building, I reported to the Taussig Cancer Center so that the radiologist and mammographer could make sure that the markers inside my breast were visible. They needed to be identified to help the doctor perform surgery on the correct areas. My mother and one of my sisters met us there. My mother led us in prayer before the nurse took me back to be checked. This procedure was comparable to a biopsy and was painful. Instead of taking the needle out of my breast, the needle stayed protruding out of my left breast as they transported me 2 buildings over to the surgical center. I was taken to pre-surgery, and my family was escorted to the waiting area and given a beeper.

After pre-surgery, I was taken to the operating room. I was greeted by the surgeons, doctors, nurses, and residents. They told me what they would be doing during surgery. The lead surgeon, who was also my breast surgeon, gave me a complete overview of what was going to occur and his expected outcomes. Everyone was positive and upbeat, which made me feel comfortable and relaxed. One nurse attempted to start the line for an IV but failed after 2 painful attempts. A more seasoned nurse started the line on the first attempt with minimal pain. The anesthesiologist explained that the medicine he was injecting into the IV would make me sleep throughout the surgery and that he would be there the entire time to monitor me. He told me to start counting backward from 100, but I don't remember counting past 97.

When I woke up in the recovery room, I was tightly bandaged around both breasts and my back. The nurse said that my surgery went well and that the lead surgeon would be in to speak with me. She asked if I were in pain. When I said that I was, she left and returned with medication that she injected into the IV. They allowed Omar to come into the recovery room. He was glad to see me and gave me a light hug because of the bandages. I stayed in recovery for about 30 minutes before being transported to another area where my entire family was able to visit.

I was relieved that this was over and patiently waited for the doctor. He arrived shortly after and reiterated that the 3-hour surgery went well. He stated that from what he could see, none of the tissue in or around the high-risk area looked cancerous. Even though I couldn't move, I started praising God with my words! My family praised God, too, and thanked the doctor for all he'd done. He stated that the tissue was sent to pathology, and he'd have the results for my follow-up appointment scheduled for May 9.

Christopher's meet and greet with the teachers and the bus ride was also scheduled for May 9. I had to choose either to reschedule my appointment or for him not to attend the meet and greet at his new school. I figured he could meet his teachers another time, but I couldn't chance missing my appointment with the surgeon. We traveled to Cleveland for my appointment.

I felt good about making the trip. I wasn't fearful of the unknown. During my week and a half of recovery at home, I didn't require any prescribed pain medication. I took over-the-counter Motrin®, which worked fine. I was starting to feel like myself laughing, smiling, talking, and enjoying life! This was the best I'd felt during this entire ordeal. It also felt good to know that this was my only appointment with the breast surgeon.

After we arrived at the clinic, I checked in and was quickly called back. Omar and I went into the room with the nurse. She clarified some information and left to get the doctor. He came in, shook our hands, and said, "Congratulations! No cancer was found in the area of concern or the tissue around it." I said, "Thank You, God. You are so awesome!"

The doctor checked the area where he'd performed surgery. There was no infection, and the area was healing nicely. He advised that I should come to an appointment that he had scheduled for August 15 with a geneticist. I'd meet with the doctor to create a plan to monitor my health if I was going to continue coming to the clinic. He explained that this was necessary because of the positive CHEK2 gene mutation. I heartily agreed.

I felt the weight of stress being lifted from my mind, and I was eager to tell the rest of my family sitting in the waiting area. I had just been given a new lease on life.

−13−

LIVE YOUR PURPOSE

As I reflect on my life, one Bible verse has been constant in my spirit: "And he rose, and rebuked the wind, and said unto the sea. Peace, be still. And the wind ceased, and there was a great calm" (Mark 4:39 KJV). It seemed like the more hell that came into my life, the more God stepped in to manage it. He saw purpose in me and didn't allow the enemy to steal my joy or my mind! But for me to hear His voice, I had to be still and go through my storms in peace. It was up to me to understand, live, and share my purpose.

I was empowered by God to be a blessing to others—to share my testimonies and experiences to help others all over the world. This assignment meant I'd have to leave my comfort zone to get the message out that *all* women must be screened for breast cancer at an earlier age. Most health insurers don't cover mammograms for women until they've reached 40 years of age and beyond, unless there is a family history.

There isn't a lot of available research for women who get breast cancer before the age of 40. From my independent study, I've discovered that early detection has saved more lives of women who were initially diagnosed with breast cancer *under* age 40. I'm a living witness that this is true. I didn't have a family history of breast cancer when I was diagnosed 17 years ago. I felt lumps in my right breast and became terrified to the extent that I didn't want to go to the doctor to get the lumps checked. I figured it was nothing, and if it was something, I didn't want to know. The devil knew God's plan for my life and didn't want to see it manifest. He knew I'd help others and give God the praise, which would draw them closer to Him. With strong faith and excellent support, I was able to conquer the fear and go to the doctor.

I want to encourage women of every age to make their health a priority. We are always concerned about taking care of others before we embrace self-love and self-care. But, if your health fails because you refused to take care of you, who will take care of your family and loved ones?

Being a woman who specializes in personal development, leadership, and relationship coaching, I am often asked how I find time to take care of myself. I'm honest with people, saying that I've always taken care of myself, but usually when I've felt extreme stress. When I encountered my battle with cancer in my 30s, I decided to take care of me since God had already done His part. My self-care consists of monthly massages, weekly exercise, traveling, and having quiet time to reflect and refocus my goals. This doesn't always work out because I have a family, but I've learned to be more deliberate about making time for me.

Everyone on earth has a purpose. The goal is to find your purpose and live it, whatever that means to you. The first part of finding your purpose is realizing who you are as a person—not who you were told you were by your parents, siblings, friends, or co-workers. I mean, knowing the inner core of who you truly are. When you reach this goal, it will be easier to find your purpose and live it regardless of other people's opinions. You will find that layers of feeling that you're not good enough—self-doubt, depression, lack of self-confidence, lack of self-worth, anxiety, and the doormat syndrome, to name a few—will peel off and prepare you for your new skin. Once you've found your purpose, there's no turning back! You'll enjoy and relish those moments spent with yourself. Should you begin to feel low, look up and know that God hasn't brought you this far to leave you. Be yourself—the person no one else can be!

CONCLUSION

Our rights as women are continuously tested. This isn't because we don't have something to say that will add value to any topic, but because for so long we've been encouraged to be seen and not heard!

As I reflect on situations that I've been through dealing with my health and now my career, I realize that I've allowed my voice to be given a back seat to other people's thoughts and opinions. Today, I know that no one's voice is more significant than mine when dealing with my issues! It's essential to be my own advocate and speak my truth. It's equally as important to ask questions when the outcome will affect me.

It wasn't a good feeling being terminated from my job, especially when there were no adequate grounds for dismissal. Be careful when people continue to smile and lie to your face, and you know their true intent. As stated in John 10:10 (ESV): "The thief comes only to steal and kill and destroy. I came that they may have life and have it abundantly." This verse reminds me that people will do and say anything to get what they want regardless of who it hurts. I've decided to use my voice and not let people steal my joy or hurt my family or me for their gain!

I've prayed about how I should take my place and use my voice to empower women in every aspect of their lives, especially when it comes to their health, mental well-being, and discrimination in the workplace. I've sat back and watched destructive things happen to other women and myself but lacked the courage to stand up. I'm no longer that person who fears what others may say, do, and think. I choose to stand up in the middle of my trials and tribulations and speak empowerment and truth at any cost.

I want to encourage all women to make sure that your rights are respected. If something is unclear, please ask clarifying questions without feeling embarrassment and shame. One of my favorite Bible verses is Proverbs 3:5-6 (KJV): "Trust in the LORD with all thine heart; and lean not unto thine own understanding. In all thy ways acknowledge him, and he shall direct thy paths." Don't be afraid to be strong and gain your voice even when the outcome doesn't seem favorable. I challenge you to have faith and understand that God is in control.

Lisa A. McDonald is a person of faith, hope, and strength. She is a motivational writer and speaker. Her courageous story of survival resonates with people who have been in challenging situations and need guidance to begin their process of healing. She shares her story of survival with boldness and truth.

Lisa has been an educator for over 23 years as a science teacher, mentor, and coach with the Sandusky (OH) City Schools and as vice-principal and principal with the Cleveland (OH) Metropolitan School District and Newark (NJ) Public Schools. She is a relationship and personal development coach, helping people all over the country realize and reach their full potential to live more prosperous lives. She is the owner of IMPAC Coaching and Consulting Group, which engages individuals, small groups, and corporate clients.

As a 17-year breast cancer survivor, Lisa is a strong advocate for early detection and mammograms for all women but with an emphasis on women under age 40. She empowers women to be vocal about their health and their wealth, helping them to realize that what they have to offer is valuable.

Lisa is honored to be the wife of Omar Sr. and the proud mother of Quincee, Omar Jr., and Christopher.

To contact the author,
please visit www.lisaamcdonald.com